ECG Interpretation

&

Rhythm Recognition

by

Jamie Bisson

(Dip. H.Sc., Dip N.Sc., Bsc. (Hons.) Crit. Care)

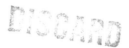

Table of Contents

Foreword

I am a clinical nurse specialist working in a major tertiary referral centre within Australia. I qualified in 1998 and since then I have been working in critical care, more specifically in a coronary care unit, cardiac high dependency units, cardiothoracic intensive care units, a paediatric and a general intensive care unit. In addition to this I have worked as an educator in all of my places of work.

I believe that ECG interpretation is a relatively simple task which can be taught to anyone given the right instruction and information. Whether you are studying for an assignment, working in critical care, or just wanting to further your knowledge then this simple e-book will teach you exactly what you need to know in an easy to understand step by step process. The examples of specific rhythm strips and ECGs will be given with reference to actual ECG's so there will not need to be any guesswork on your behalf.

This ebook is not necessarily designed to provide extensive explanation for the specific rhythms and ECG's, it was made for identification purposes only.

Basic Rhythm strip analysis

Normal Sinus Rhythm

Before we start to analyse any ECG we need to establish what a basic rhythm looks like. The basic rhythm is normal sinus rhythm, which consists of a P-wave, QRS complex and a T wave.

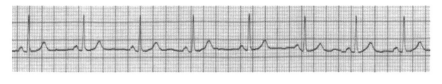

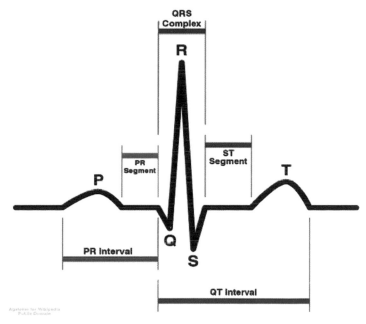

The P wave represents atrial depolarisation, or electrical firing.

The QRS complex represents ventricular depolarisation, or electrical firing. The normal width of this complex is less than 3 small squares, which is 0.12 seconds.

The T wave represents ventricular re-polarisation, or getting the cells ready for another depolarisation.

The PR interval is the time interval between the P wave and the onset of the QRS, which reflects the time between sino-atrial (SA) node and ventricular depolarisation. Normal duration is between 3 and 5 small squares (0.12 - 0.2 seconds).

The SA node is responsible for (in normal sinus rhythm) atrial depolarisation. The AV node (in normal sinus rhythm) initiates ventricular depolarisation.

To read the rhythm strip you need to, as with most things, follow a systematic approach. The method of analysis that I advocate is the following:

1:          Is there a P wave?

2:          Is there a QRS complex?

3:          Is there a T wave?

4:          Is the rhythm regular?

5:          Is the rhythm regularly regular (with that I mean is there a regular pattern that the potentially irregular rhythm follows)?

With normal sinus rhythm there is a P wave, a QRS complex, and a T wave. The rhythm is regular, and it is regularly regular.

Normal sinus rhythm generally is at a rate of between 60 and 100 beats per minute. To establish the rate of the rhythm, count the number of large squares between the point, for example R to R, and divide this into 300. To demonstrate this with the prior example, there are almost 4 large squares between R points, therefore 300 ÷ 4 = 75 beats per minute.

An important note when analysing a rhythm strip is that whenever you are unsure if there is a T wave, if you see another QRS complex then there must have been a T wave. This is because without a T wave there would be no further ventricular depolarisation or electrical firing. The reason for this is that the myocardial cells need to reach the correct electrical charge to fire again.

Sinus bradycardia

This rhythm is the same as normal sinus rhythm, however the rate is less than 60 beats per minute.

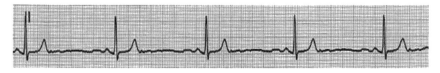

Sinus tachycardia

This rhythm is the same as normal sinus rhythm, but the rate is greater than 100 beats per minute.

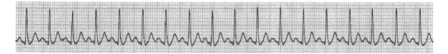

Atrial Fibrillation

Atrial fibrillation simply refers to the atria fibrillating, or quivering. Atrial fibrillation is characterised by a lack of definitive P waves. The QRS complexes and T waves will be present, however the rate of the rhythm will be irregular, generally somewhere between 120 to 160 beats per minute. It is however possible for atrial fibrillation to be slower than 120 beats per minute, however it is less common. Slow atrial fibrillation can range from rates between 50 and 120 beats per minute.

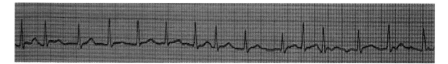

So, to follow the method I advocate: there are no definitive P waves, there are QRS complexes, and T waves; the rhythm is irregular and it is irregularly irregular.

Actual fibrillation is a phenomenon where an overexcited area of the atria is firing at anywhere around 300 beats per minute. Although the atria are firing at this rate the AV node will not allow all the impulses to depolarise the ventricles. The atrial activity does not look like normal P waves as the electrical impulse is originating from somewhere within the atria and not following the normal conduction pathway.

The normal conduction pathway originates from the SA node to the AV node, down the Bundle of His, bundle branches and through to the Purkinje fibres. The normal conduction pathway consists of myelinated fibres which transmit impulses at incredibly fast speeds. This is displayed by narrow complexes, for example the QRS complex within 3 small squares or 0.12 seconds. If an impulse originates outside of the normal conduction pathway the complexes would be broad and bizarre in appearance. In atrial fibrillation the atrial activity is so fast that it may not be seen on the ECG and if it is seen they resemble nothing like the normal P waves. In fact these atrial depolarisation's are generally referred to as f waves.

Atrial flutter

Atrial flutter is a rhythm that has definite P waves (which in atrial flutter are actually referred to as F waves) which are saw–tooth in appearance. There are QRS complexes and T waves. The ventricular rhythm may be regular or irregular.

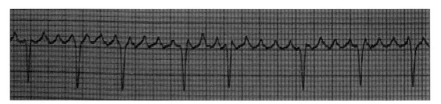

Intrinsically with atrial flutter, again there is over–excitation of the atria. However, differing from atrial fibrillation, atrial flutter is where the atria are depolarising continuously and regularly which gives the saw-tooth appearance.

Atrial ectopics / Supra-ventricular extrasystole

Atrial ectopics are early beats that originate from the atria. Basically what you will see is a P wave that is not exactly the same shape as the other P waves, that comes earlier in the rhythm than expected, followed by a QRS, T wave and then a compensatory pause. Because they originate from within the atria and not from the

SA node they will take longer to depolarise the atria and as such the shape will be broader than normal - although it may not be a noticeable widening. In the following example, the P wave is actually hidden in the R wave (the first initial upward deflection in the QRS).

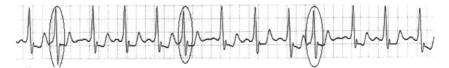

Ventricular Ectopics / Ventricular extrasystole

Ventricular ectopics are simply early ventricular beats which do not originate from the AV node; as such the depolarisation takes longer and the QRS is therefore wider (>0.12 seconds or 3 small squares) and more bizarre in its morphology. The patient may, or may not, have a pulse with the ventricular ectopic. In the following example if this ectopic or extrasystole occurs again and is the same shape it would be called mono or uni-focal in origin.

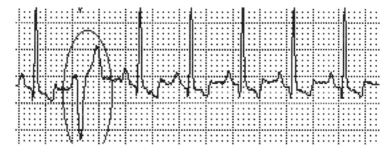

Polymorphic or multifocal ventricular ectopics / extrasystoles

These are ventricular pre-excitations which occur from differing areas of the ventricles. The QRS is again broad and bizarre when the ectopic/extrasystole occurs, but they are different shapes, as the depolarisation is originating from differing areas of the ventricles, as is shown in the following example.

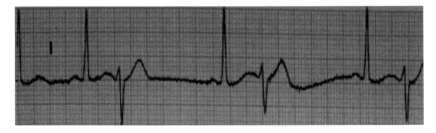

Bigeminy

Bigeminy is shown on a rhythm strip as an intrinsic beat, followed with an ectopic/extrasystole and then an intrinsic beat; this pattern continues. The following example shows the patient's intrinsic sinus rhythm with ventricular ectopics/extrasystoles. The patient may, or may not have a pulse with the ectopic/extrasystole.

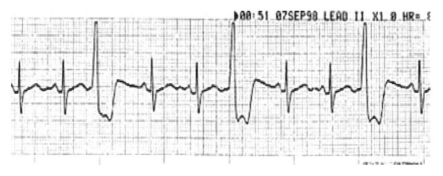

Trigeminy

Trigeminy is simply 2 intrinsic beats followed by an ectopic/extrasystole. The patient may, or may not have a pulse with the ectopic/extrasystole.

Courtesy of Dr Chirk Jenn Ng

Supra-ventricular tachycardia

A supra-ventricular tachycardia (SVT) is basically any tachycardia that originates from above the ventricles (hence supra), so in theory a sinus tachycardia is an SVT as the rhythm is originating from the SA node. An SVT will usually have a narrow (≤0.12 seconds or 3 small squares) QRS complex, unless the patient has a bundle branch block, or an aberrant conduction - to be discussed later. If an overexcited area of the atria are firing and then the impulse travels down the myelinated fibres; the impulse then passes through the AV node and the ventricles depolarise at a rapid rate. Because the impulse is traveling down the myelinated pathways and through the AV node the impulse is traveling very quickly, so the QRS complexes are narrow.

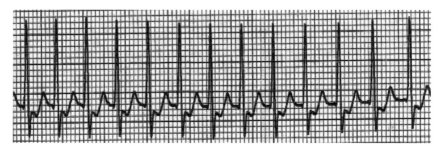

Ventricular fibrillation

Ventricular fibrillation, like a atrial fibrillation, refers to the ventricles quivering. A hugely significant difference between atrial fibrillation and ventricular fibrillation is that ventricular fibrillation is a life threatening rhythm that needs emergency treatment in the form of electrical cardioversion, cardiopulmonary resuscitation and advanced life support.

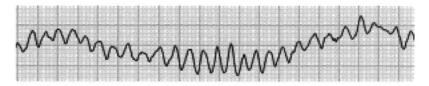

Ventricular fibrillation is shown as an unsystematic wiggling, jagged, spiky appearance. The rhythm should be confirmed by checking the ECG leads are attached properly to the patient. Giving the patient a brief but definite shake at this point would also not be frowned upon! They should be no P-wave, QRS complexes that are unrecognisable from how it should appear and no definitive T wave.

The reason ventricular fibrillation is a life-threatening rhythm is because the ventricles are the main pumping chambers within the heart and if they are made ineffective there will be no circulating volume to the rest of the body and subsequently death will follow if not rapidly treated. With atrial fibrillation the atria only supply 10-30% of the cardiac output, so if the atria are not pumping as normal the body can overcome it, however if the ventricles aren't pumping properly nothing can overcome that besides emergency lifesaving intervention.

Fine ventricular fibrillation

Fine ventricular fibrillation is exactly the same as normal ventricular fibrillation, but the size or amplitude of the ventricular rhythm is a lot smaller. It can often look like asystole when the ECG amplitude or gain is turned down. The treatment for fine ventricular fibrillation is exactly the same as normal ventricular fibrillation.

Ventricular tachycardia

Ventricular tachycardia in theory should have a P wave in it, however in practice this is hard to see. The QRS complex will be uniformly spiky, or uniformly rounded in appearance and will have a definite shape that repeats itself, which is very unlike ventricular fibrillation. There is a T wave, but again, this may not be seen. The treatment of this will depend upon whether the patient has a pulse or not.

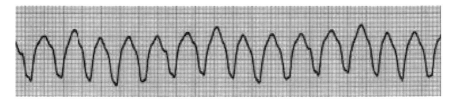

Torsades de Pointes / Polymorphic ventricular tachycardia

This looks the same a ventricular tachycardia, however the amplitude of the QRS undulates. This is due to a rotation of the electrical axis or direction of electrical impulses.

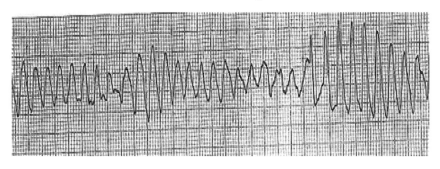

Asystole

Asystole is shown as no cardiac activity. No P, QRS or T waves. The trace is often undulating in appearance and not truly a flat line. This trace needs to be confirmed in 2 ECG leads and the amplitude, or ECG gain, should be turned right up to exclude fine ventricular fibrillation. This is another life threatening arrhythmia that requires urgent cardiopulmonary resuscitation and advanced life support.

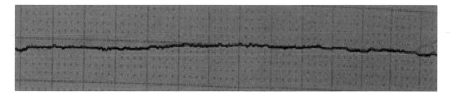

Ventricular standstill

Ventricular standstill is very similar to asystole, however there are P waves present, as shown below. Again this is a life threatening arrhythmia that requires urgent cardiopulmonary resuscitation and advanced life support +/- cardiac pacing.

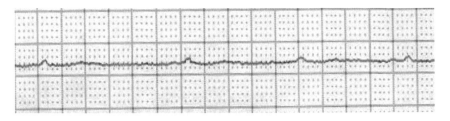

Electro-Mechanical-Dissociation / Pulseless Electrical Activity

This is another life threatening rhythm where cardiopulmonary resuscitation and advanced life support is needed. It is shown by any life sustaining rhythm, however there is no pulse associated with it. An example of this would be sinus bradycardia on the monitor accompanied by a lack of pulse.

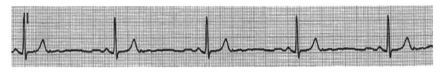

P Mitrale

P mitrale is a rhythm that is seen when there is mitral valve dysfunction, regurgitation, stenosis and potentially a general overload of the left atrium. It is shown as an M shape on the P wave, as shown below.

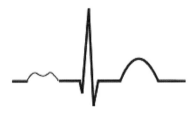

P Pulmonale

P pulmonale is a rhythm that is seen in pulmonary congestion, which when chronic causes an enlarged right atrium and tall peaked P wave, as shown below.

Heart Blocks

First degree heart block / First degree atrioventricular block

First degree heart block is very simply a lengthened PR interval greater than 5 small squares or 0.2 seconds. This rhythm is often a sign of a diseased AV node, however it is also seen in myocarditis, electrolyte disturbances and sometimes following certain drugs that increase the refractory time of the AV node (including, but not limited to calcium channel blockers and beta blockers). This rhythm is benign, however people in a first degree heart block are more likely to develop into a second degree heart block if they are given certain anti-arrhythmic medications. In the following example the first two lines show the most obvious first degree heart block.

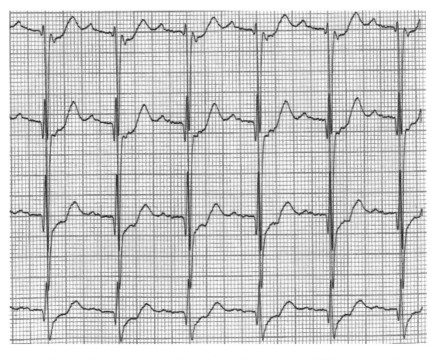

Second degree heart block mobitz type 1 / Wenckebach

Second degree heart block (type 1) is also known as Wenckebach, after its founder Karel Frederik Wenckebach in 1899. It is nearly always due to a diseased AV node. This rhythm is basically a progressive lengthening of the PR interval until there is a P wave with no QRS depolarisation followed by another P wave, a QRS complex and a T wave. The PR intervals get longer and longer until the QRS is dropped. In the following example there is a 4:1 block (4 conducted QRS beats and 1 dropped QRS beat as shown with the red circles).

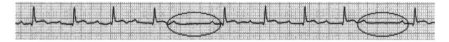

If you ever see a P wave not followed by a QRS depolarisation and another P wave, then you have a second degree heart block at the very least.

Second degree heart block mobitz type 2

With second degree heart block (type 2) there is often a normal intrinsic beat with P, QRS and T waves, followed by a P wave, no QRS and then another intrinsic beat. If this pattern continues it would be classed as a second degree heart block (type 2) with a 1:1 block. The 1:1 block refers to 1 normal beat : 1 dropped QRS.

It is however more common to see a second degree heart block (type 2) with a 2:1 (as shown below), or a 3:1 heart block. This is basically two or three normal intrinsic beats, followed by a P wave with no QRS. It then continues with the same pattern.

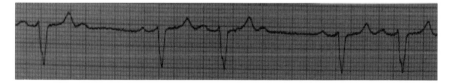

It is also possible and not too uncommon to have a second degree heart block (type 2) with a variable block. So in this instance you may have one intrinsic beat with 1 dropped QRS, followed by 3 intrinsic beats and a dropped QRS, next followed by 2 intrinsic beats and so on.

Third degree heart block / Complete heart block

This rhythm is basically a disassociation between the atria and the ventricles, where the atria will depolarise at about 60-70 beats per minute and the ventricles will beat at about 40 beats per minute. Both the atria (P waves) and the ventricles (QRS complexes) are regular in their respective rates, but they are not associated with one another; for example atria at 60beats per minute and ventricles at 40 beats per minute. The following example shows the ventricular rate at approximately 35 beats per minute in a dotted arrow and the atria at approximately 75 beats per minute in solid arrows. Note the ventricular rate and atrial rate are different. This example also shows some aberrant conduction of the ventricles as they are greater than 0.12 seconds or 3 small squares. Aberrant conduction refers to conduction that does not follow the normal pathway and as such is broad and bizarre in its appearance.

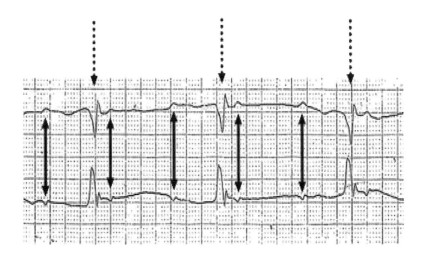

More often than not patients with this rhythm are unstable and need urgent cardiac pacing.

Wolff-Parkinson-White Syndrome

Wolff-Parkinson-White Syndrome is where there is aberrant conduction between the ventricles and atria, which can lead the ventricles to beat at a very fast rate. This aberrant conduction pathway is known as the Bundle of Kent, as shown below.

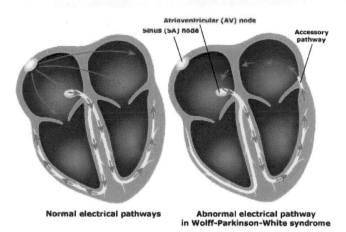

Normal electrical pathways

**Abnormal electrical pathway
in Wolff-Parkinson-White syndrome**

Wolff-Parkinson-White Syndrome is shown on the ECG as a delta wave, or slur on the R wave of the QRS. and a short PR interval, as the following example shows.

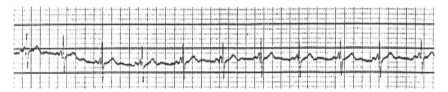

ECG Analysis

An ECG is a recording of 12 aspects of heart. When an ECG is performed it utilises 10 physical leads which are attached to the patient. The ECG machine takes 10 leads and with the help of some calculations it derives an extra 2 leads of data.

To understand this we need to explain which lead is looking at each specific region of the heart.

Limb leads

Lead I & AVL: Lateral regions of the heart

Lead II, III & AVF: Inferior regions of the heart

Chest leads

V1 & V2:   Anteroseptal region of the heart

V3 & V4:   Anterior region of the heart

V5 & V6:   Lateral region of the heart

The four limb leads look on a vertical and diagonal plain and the chest leads look on a horizontal plain through the heart, so limb lead II & III diagonally look up. Limb lead AVL & AVR look diagonally down. The RL lead is the grounding or neutral lead and no data is collected from that lead directly, it just completes the electrical circuit. Calculations are made with the limb leads to provide the extra data for limb lead I, AVF & III. This is how the ECG machine gets the extra leads, giving the 10 leads physical leads a 12 lead view. In the following image the green labels are the formulated extra leads. Please note, however that wrist and leg limb lead placement can also be used, however it will alter the ECG slightly. Some cardiologists will insist on wrist and leg placements and some will be happy with shoulder and hip placement; consistency is the key here in using the ECG in a fully diagnostic manner.

If an impulse is travelling towards a lead it will have a mainly positive deflection and if it is travelling away from the lead it will have a mainly negative deflection. It is important to note that all normal impulses travel away from AVR, so this lead displays negative deflecting waves. Lead II should be mainly positive in the normal patient as most of the impulse is moving towards the lead.

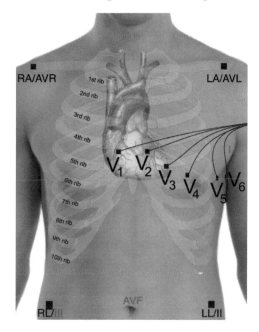

Ischaemia

Ischaemia is shown as either T wave inversion or ST depression. ST segments are defined as the area between the J and T point. ST segments should follow the isoelectric line and should therefore not be elevated or depressed in the normal person. The following example shows ST elevation.

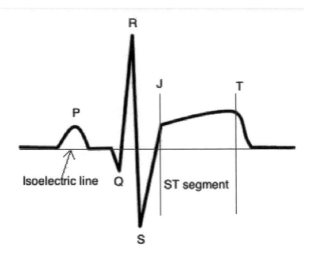

Next shows an ECG with mainly anterolateral ischaemia with T wave inversion.

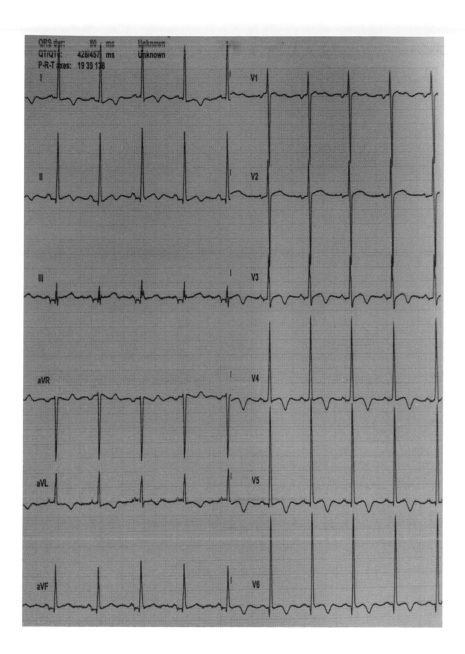
QRS dur: 80   ms   Unknown
QT/QTc: 428/457   ms   Unknown
P-R-T axes: 19 39 138

I   V1

II   V2

III   I   V3

aVR   I   V4

aVL   I   V5

aVF   I   V6

The following ECG shows ST depression in the anterolateral leads.

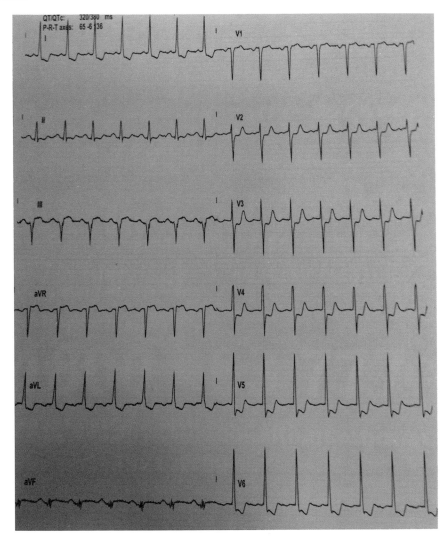

ST elevation

ST elevation is often due to an acute myocardial infarction, however it can also be due to coronary artery spasm. This is why when someone presents with ST elevation the idea is to try some nitrates to see if the patient becomes pain-free and the ST segments normalise.

A myocardial infarction is shown on the ECG as 1 mm ST elevation in 2 or more limb leads and 2 mm ST elevation in 2 or more chest leads.

Remember however, that a myocardial infarction is not diagnosed by ECG alone, it is diagnosed by patient history, description of symptoms, cardiac enzymes and their ECG. The ultimate diagnosis of a myocardial infarction is made with a cardiac angiogram where radiographic contrast is injected into the coronary arteries to visualise any narrowing (potential for ischaemia) or blockages (acute or chronic infarctions).

Development of a full thickness / transmural myocardial infarction

A full thickness / transmural myocardial infarction progresses on the ECG as follows. Please note that the times are approximate and depend upon a number of factors:

Onset: ST elevation of more than 2 mm on 2 or more chest leads or 1 mm in 2 or more limb leads.

Within 6hrs Development of q waves (q waves are a small negative deflection from the Q point, which are less than a 3rd of the R wave)

Within 12 hrs Development of Q waves (Q waves are defined as a negative deflection from the Q point greater than a 3rd of the R wave)

At 24 hours: Q waves, ST segments which are flat, along with flat or biphasic (half up and half down) T waves

At 48 hours: Q waves with deeply inverted T waves

At 4 days: Q waves with normal T waves

The example below shows the development without Q waves, so this infarct was not a full thickness or transmural myocardial infarction, but instead a sub-endocardial, or partial thickness myocardial infarction.

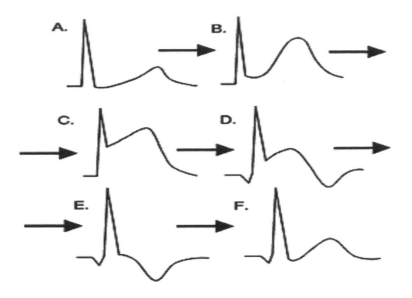

Please note that limb lead III often has a Q wave in it, which is not a sign of an old infarct, as will chest lead V1 & V2, especially if their placement on the patients chest is a bit high (most of the impulse is moving away from the leads).

Sub-endocardial myocardial infarction

A sub-endocardial myocardial infarction can be shown as T wave inversion on the ECG and can look exactly the same as T wave inversion ischaemia, or it may also present with ST elevation. The following example shows a global sub-endocardial myocardial infarction. The key with a sub-endocardial or partial thickness myocardial infarction is that there are no Q waves present after the infarct. It may appear that chest leads V2 and V3 have Q waves, however on closer inspection there is a small upward deflection before the negative deflection, so this negative deflection would be called an S wave, as it came after the r wave (not capital R, as it is a small wave).

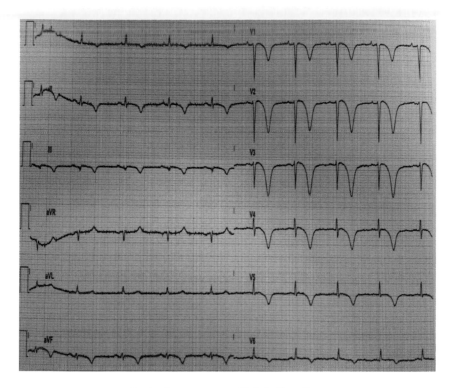

<u>Anterior myocardial infarction</u>

The ECG will show with ST elevation in the anterior region of the heart (chest leads V1 - V4), there may also often be reciprocal changes, or ST depression, in the inferior regions (limb leads II, III & AVF). Depending on how extensive the infarct is there may also be ST elevation in V5 & V6.

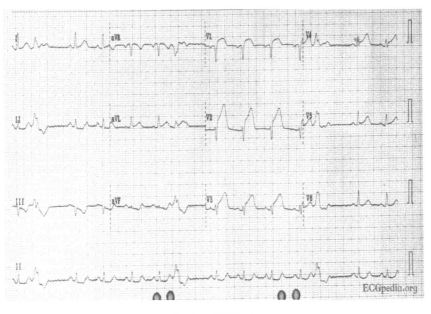

Inferior myocardial infarction

This myocardial infarction will be shown on the ECG as ST elevation in the inferior regions (II, III & AVF), as shown in the following ECG. Often there are lateral reciprocal changes, or ST depression, in limb leads I, AVL and possibly V5 – V6.

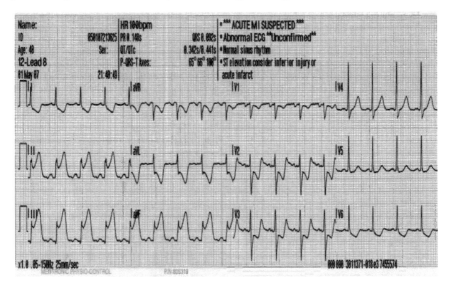

Posterior myocardial infarction

It is not uncommon that when there is an inferior myocardial infarction, as with the identical prior and next ECG there is also posterior involvement, which is shown as ST depression in leads V1 - V3.

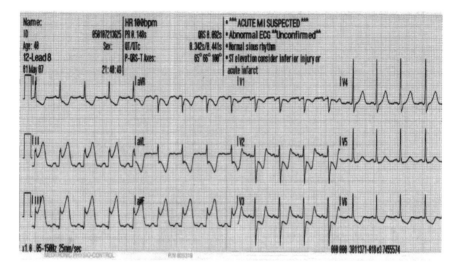

To detect larger posterior infarcts chest leads V4 - 6 are removed and placed in the same position, but on the back of the patient on the left hand side. These new chest leads and called V7 - 9. Along with the posterior involvement there is also a higher probability of right ventricular infarction. This is detected by mirroring the chest lead placements on the right side of the chest, leaving V1 & V2 in their normal place. These new leads should be referred to as V3R - V6R to identify the leads as right sided. With posterior and right sided myocardial infarctions only 1 mm of ST elevation is needed to gain ECG significance in the chest leads.

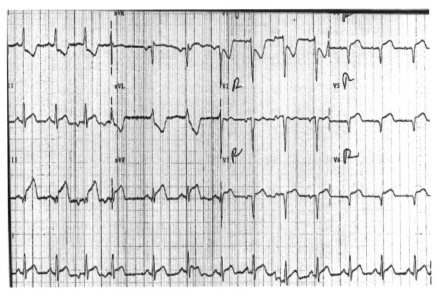

Infero-lateral myocardial infarction

This is displayed as ST elevation in the inferior regions and the lateral regions (II, III, AVF, I, AVL and possibly V5 - 6). The following example also has some anterior involvement as can be seen with ST elevation in V3 and V4. A purely infero-lateral myocardial infarction, however only has ST elevation in leads II, III, AVF, I, AVL and possibly V5 and V6.

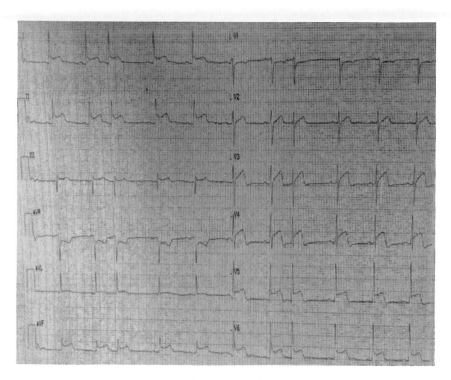

<u>Anterolateral myocardial infarction</u>

Shown on the ECG as ST elevation in the anterior and lateral leads (V3 - V6, I, AVL and possibly V1 - 2).

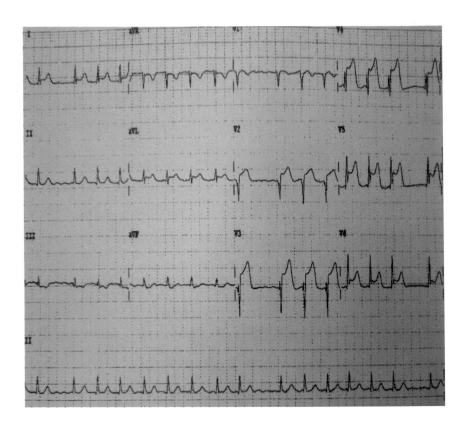

Conduction issues

The following section covers ECG's that are present when there are problems with the hearts native conduction system. Below is an image of the heart with the associated conduction structures:

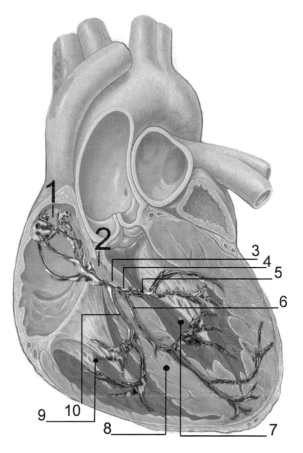

1:   SA node

2:   AV node

3:   Bundle of His

4:   Left bundle branch

5:   Left posterior fascicle

6:          Left anterior fascicle

7:          Left ventricle

8:          Ventricular septum

9:          Right ventricle

10:         Right bundle branch

Left bundle branch block

This morphology happens because the left bundle branch is unable to conduct impulses. Bundle branch blocks are easy to remember. If you can remember the words "william" and "marrow" you will be half way there. Very basically, with a left bundle branch block there is a "W" shape in V1 and an "M" shape in V6 - hence "William". The morphology does not exactly follow an M or W shape, but comes close. To be more precise there is a QS or rS in V1 and a RsR in V6. The non-capital letters reflect a small wave and the capital letters refer to large waves. Bundle branch blocks must have a QRS which is greater than 3 small squares or 0.12 seconds. Left bundle branch blocks are serious: if they are new then it is very possible that the patient is having a myocardial infarction. However it may also be due to aortic stenosis and dilated cardiomyopathies. The following example shows a left bundle branch block with atrial ectopics. Some authors believe that if you have a left bundle branch block you therefore have a bifascicular block (bifascicular blocks will be described later).

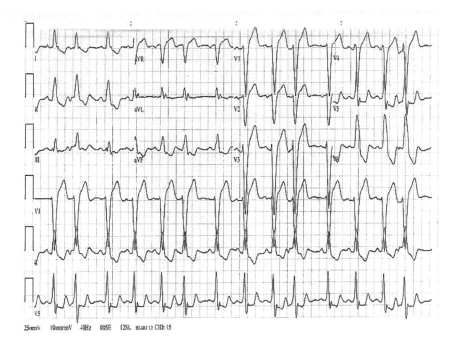

Right bundle branch block

With the right bundle branch block there is a "M" shape in V1 and a "W" shape in V6. To be more precise in the morphology of the right bundle branch block an rSR is seen in V1 and qRS in V6. Remember that the QRS must be greater than 0.12 seconds or 3 small squares. Right bundle branch blocks are benign in their ECG alone. A right bundle branch block is often present when increased right sided heart pressures are present, for example with a pulmonary embolism, hypertension, cardiomyopathies, congenital heart disease and trauma to the right ventricle. Again the M and W shape are not exact, but come close.

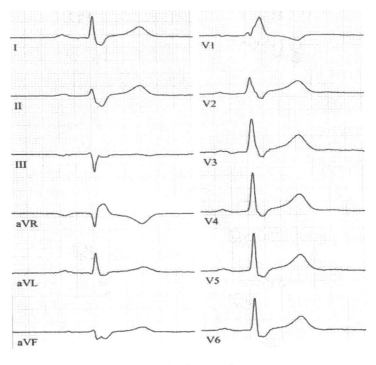

Ventricular pacing

Ventricular pacing is shown on the ECG as a pacing spike at the Q point, followed by a broad and bizarre QRS as the depolarisation does not follow the normal conduction pathways. In the following example the pacing spikes can clearly be seen in V2 - V6.

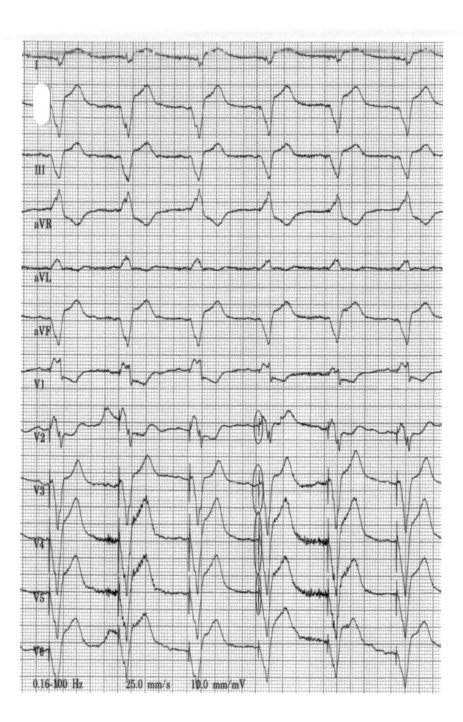

Atrial pacing

Atrial pacing is shown on the ECG as a pacing spike at the P point, followed by a broad and bizarre P wave as the depolarisation does not follow the normal conduction pathway. The different morphology of the paced P wave may not be that noticeable, but the spikes will be.

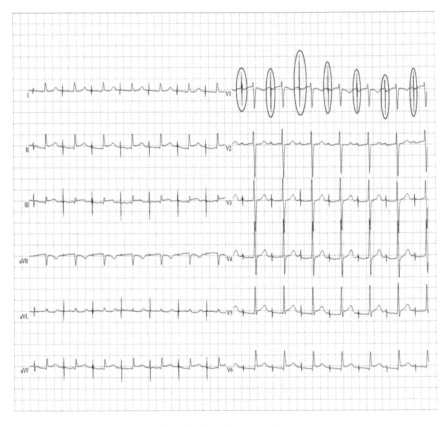

Dual chamber pacing

With dual chamber pacing (atria and ventricles), pacing spikes will be seen before the P wave and at the Q point with broad and bizarre waves being produced. In the following example pacing spikes can clearly be seen in V3, V4 and limb lead III that clearly identify atrial and ventricular pacing.

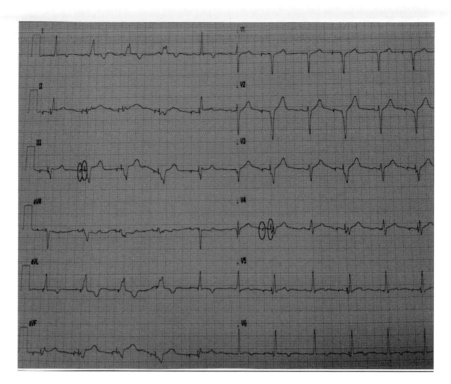

Axis deviation

To find out the axis deviation on an ECG there are many ways of doing it, but the easiest way that I teach is to plot a vertical line on the ECG paper 10 mm long and a horizontal line 10 mm long in the middle of the vertical line. Write "I" on the right of the horizontal line and "AVF" on the bottom of the vertical line. From the isoelectric line of limb lead I, count the number of small squares the QRS has an upward deflection and then subtract that number by the number of small squares the QRS deviates down from the isoelectric line. Plot the number on the ECG paper, either towards (making it a positive number) or away from the "I" mark (making it a negative number). Then do the same with limb lead AVF. Now join the two marks on the ECG paper and draw a line from the centre to the intersecting point from the two marks. An example is shown next:

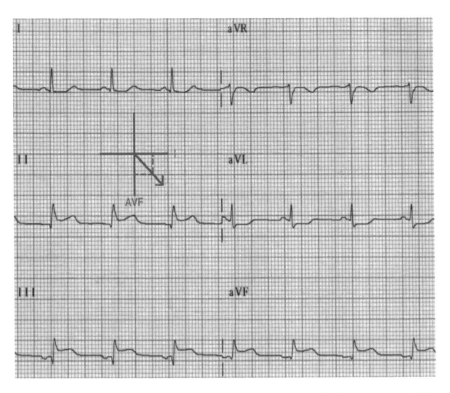

If the line marked "I" is known as 0° and AVF is known as +90°, normal axis is defined as -30° to +90°. Right axis deviation is in the regions of +90° to +180°. Left axis deviation is defined as -30° to -90°.

Bifascicular block

Bifascicular block is defined as a right bundle branch block with either a left or right axis deviation. In this pattern the ventricles are depolarised with the one remaining fascicle, either the left anterior fascicle or the left posterior fascicle. If the left anterior fascicle is blocked then a left axis deviation will be present, but if the left posterior fascicle is blocked then there will be a right axis deviation. A bifascicular block affecting the left anterior fascicle is the most common type of bifascicular block, as shown next. People who have a bifascicular block are more likely to develop a trifascicular block and complete heart block.

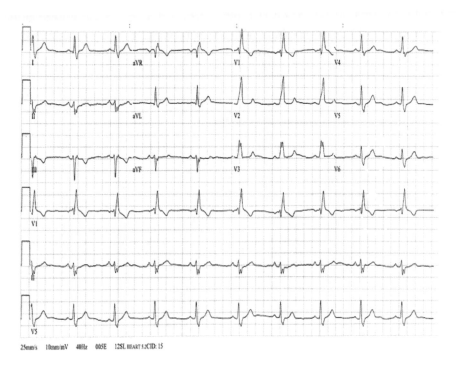

25mm/s 10mm/mV 40Hz 005E 12SL HEART 5.2CID: 15

Incomplete Trifascicular block

This is diagnosed on an ECG as either a:

1:          Right bundle branch block with a first degree heart block and a left or right axis deviation (this is the most common type of trifascicular block);

2:          Right bundle branch block with a second degree heart block and a left or right axis deviation;

3:          Right bundle branch block with alternating left and right axis.

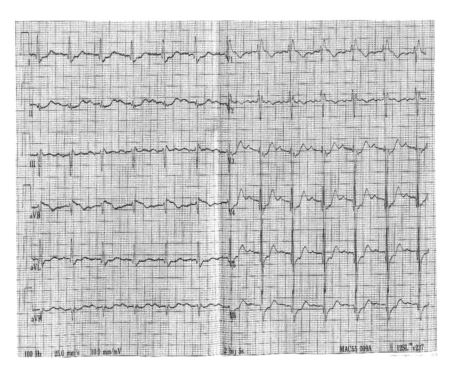

Complete Trifascicular block

This is defined on an ECG as complete heart block with a right bundle branch block and either a left or right axis deviation.

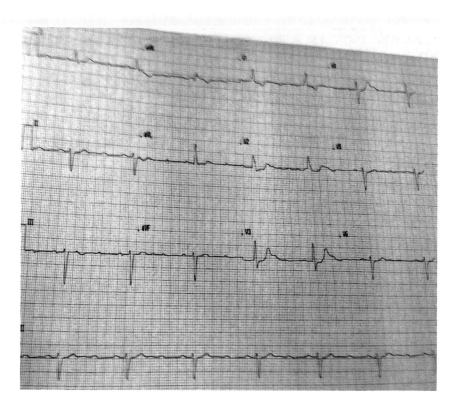

Acknowledgements

I would like to thank the following people and organisations for their kind donations of a couple of the ECG's used in this ebook:

Dr Peter Fletcher, Cardiologist, John Hunter Hospital, Newcastle, NSW, Australia

Dr Chirk Jenn Ng, Associate Professor, Faculty of Medicine, University of Malaya, Kuala Lumpur, Malaysia

ECGpedia

Dr Cafer Zorkun, Cardiologist, Yedikule Education & Research Hospital, Istanbul, Turkey

Made in the USA
San Bernardino, CA
23 September 2013